I0493911

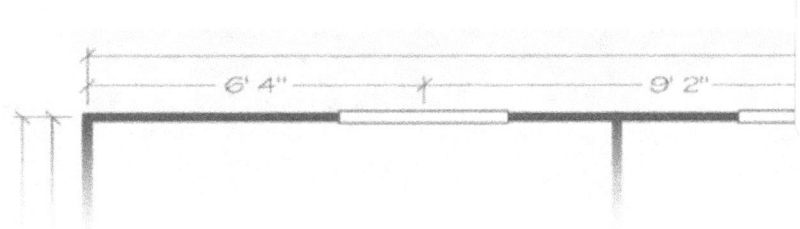

Evaluation Toolkit
for Smoke-Free Policies

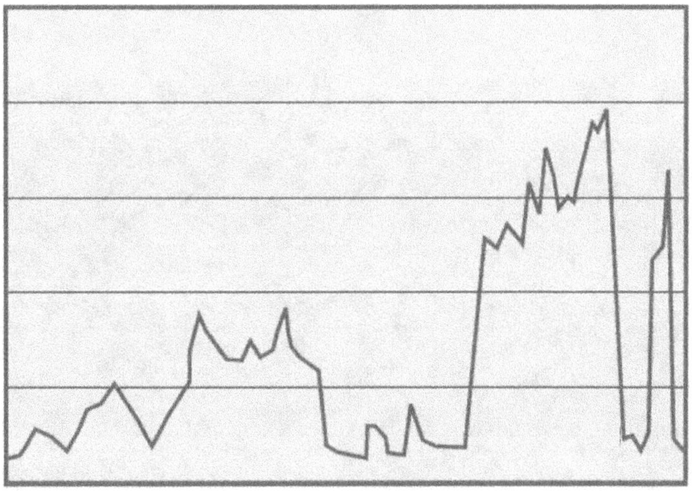

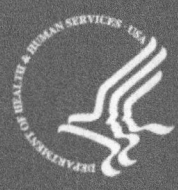

U.S. DEPARTMENT OF HEALTH AND HUMAN SERVICES
CENTERS FOR DISEASE CONTROL AND PREVENTION

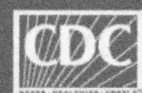

We would like to thank the New York State Tobacco Control Program, which pioneered several of the evaluation approaches reviewed in this publication, for its generosity in sharing its evaluation strategy and its study protocols. We would also like to acknowledge ClearWay Minnesota's *A Toolkit for Implementing and Defending Smoke-Free Ordinances*, which helped us in organizing and presenting the information in this publication.

Ordering Information
To download or order copies of this book, go to http://www.cdc.gov/tobacco to order single copies, or call toll-free
1 (800) CDC-INFO
1 (800) 232-4636

Centers for Disease Control and Prevention. *Evaluation Toolkit for Smoke-Free Policies*. Atlanta: U.S. Department of Health and Human Services; 2008. Available at http://www.cdc.gov/tobacco.

Evaluation Toolkit

for

Smoke-Free Policies

Brett Loomis, MS
Matthew Farrelly, PhD
Joanne Pais, MS
RTI International

Andrew Hyland, PhD
Roswell Park Cancer Institute

Paul Mowery, MA
Biostatistics, Inc.

Stephen Babb, MPH
Natasha Jamison, MPH
Jerelyn Jordan, BA
CDC Office on Smoking and Health

U.S. DEPARTMENT OF HEALTH AND HUMAN SERVICES
Centers for Disease Control and Prevention
Coordinating Center for Health Promotion
National Center for Chronic Disease Prevention and Health Promotion
Office on Smoking and Health

Contents

INTRODUCTION

This publication is intended for use by Centers for Disease Control and Prevention (CDC) staff in providing technical assistance to state tobacco control programs on approaches to evaluating the effects of state policies and laws that restrict smoking in workplaces and public places. (These policies and laws are often referred to as "smoke-free" policies and laws.) Additionally, it is intended for use by state tobacco control program evaluation staff in conducting such evaluations, and for use by national tobacco control partner organizations and other public health professionals in responding to requests for technical assistance on this topic.

This publication can also be used by state tobacco control program staff to help community tobacco control programs and coalitions assess the impact of local smoke-free laws. The evaluation approaches described in this publication and the findings of studies conducted using these approaches may also be useful to other stakeholders who are interested in the effects of smoke-free laws, including business organizations (e.g., chambers of commerce, restaurant associations) and labor unions. This publication is based on the science reviewed in the 2006 U.S. Surgeon General's Report, on more recent published studies, and on the experiences of U.S. states and other countries that have implemented and evaluated smoke-free laws.

Increasingly, states and communities are passing laws to make indoor workplaces and public places, including restaurants and bars, smoke-free. Once a smoke-free law is passed, state and local tobacco control programs and their stakeholders often want to evaluate the law's effects to assess if the law is achieving its intended benefits and to be certain that it is not having negative side effects. An evaluation can also help answer questions that policy makers and other key stakeholders may have about a law's impact.

In most cases, evaluation results are likely to indicate that a smoke-free law is having effects that are broadly similar to those observed in other sites. Nevertheless, confirming that this is the case is important for local evaluation and surveillance purposes and for responding to the questions and interests of stakeholders, who typically want to review local data. In other cases, evaluations may bring to light different or unexpected findings that may be helpful in identifying gaps or deficiencies in the law (e.g., exemptions for certain venues), in the implementation and enforcement of the law, or in the process leading to the enactment and implementation of the law (e.g., inadequate education of the public and the business community).

Evaluation results may also be useful in comparing the effects of smoke-free laws in different sites (e.g., sites with more comprehensive laws compared with sites with less comprehensive laws, urban compared with rural sites, sites with different population compositions, state laws compared with local laws, state laws in states with previous experience with local smoke-free laws compared with state laws in states without such experience).

Evaluating a smoke-free law involves considerable planning before the law takes effect. One major reason is that several of the evaluation studies commonly used require the collection of baseline, pre-implementation data. Additionally, gathering data before a law is passed may be necessary to demonstrate the need for a law.

Several factors should be considered to determine what studies to undertake:

- The stage the site has reached in the policy process.

- The types of information that policy makers, the news media, the business community, and the public are requesting.

- The provisions of the law, including any exemptions, and the venues that the law does and does not cover.

- The resources available to evaluate the law.

Most sites will not need to conduct all the studies described in this document. Sites should make strategic decisions about which studies to undertake on the basis of their local situations, needs, and resources. The *Evaluation Toolkit for Smoke-Free Policies* is designed to help state and local tobacco control programs select the specific studies that are best suited to their needs and resources. It also provides general information on how to design and conduct each study.

Studies of smoke-free laws typically examine one of five outcomes: public support, compliance, air quality, employee health, and economic impact. Section 1 of this publication outlines four major issues to consider when selecting among these studies. Section 2 provides an overview of the studies, including what information the studies generate, how this information can be used, what potential pitfalls to guard against, when to collect data, and what specific approaches are available. Section 3, which is primarily intended for staff in CDC's Office on Smoking and Health and others who provide technical assistance to state and local tobacco control programs, draws on the criteria in Section 1 to present a step-by-step process to help programs decide which studies are most appropriate for their site. Finally, Section 4 provides a selected bibliography of key peer-reviewed studies for each of the five types of studies examined.

CHOOSING AMONG EVALUATION STUDIES FOR SMOKE-FREE POLICIES

There are five broad studies that state or local tobacco control programs can conduct to prepare for a smoke-free law or to evaluate the law's effects after its implementation. Most sites will not need to conduct all five studies. Each site should decide which studies best meet its needs and can be implemented feasibly with its resources. The purpose of this section is to discuss several factors that sites should consider when developing an evaluation plan for a smoke-free law. After reading this section, a decision maker should understand how the local context—including the stage the site has reached in the policy process; the kinds of information that are being requested by policy makers, the news media, the business community, and the public; the specific provisions of the law in question; and the resources available to a site—helps determine what outcomes to assess. Section 2 provides greater detail on the five types of studies.

The five types of studies are as follows:

- **Public Support.** These studies use surveys to assess public awareness of the health effects of secondhand smoke and of the proposed policy and public support for smoke-free environments and for a smoke-free law. They are useful before a law has been passed to determine if support is sufficiently high to warrant moving forward and to document the levels of support. After a law has been passed and implemented, these studies track levels of support and changes in these levels over time.

- **Compliance.** These studies are useful for assessing compliance with a smoke-free law in hospitality venues and other workplaces and public places. They can be used to document compliance rates, to assess how implementation is proceeding, to identify types of venues and geographic regions where increased educational and enforcement efforts are needed, and to monitor trends in compliance over time.

- **Air Quality Monitoring.** These studies use a small, portable device to measure particulate matter suspended in air. The study results can be used before a law takes effect to document air quality in hospitality venues that allow smoking. After a law has taken effect, these studies can be used to assess changes in air quality in these venues.

- **Employee Health.** These studies can be used before a law takes effect to assess secondhand smoke exposure and related health problems among nonsmoking employees in hospitality venues that allow smoking. After a law has been implemented, these studies can measure changes that occur in employees' secondhand smoke exposure and related health outcomes. For employee health studies, it is critical to collect data before and after the law goes into effect.

- **Economic Impact.** These studies use objective data on employment levels and taxable sales revenues to assess the economic impact of a smoke-free law on hospitality venues such as restaurants, bars, and casinos.

The last three types of studies typically focus on hospitality venues, while the first two study types are also applicable to other workplaces and public places.

In addition to these five types of studies, several studies have examined the impact of smoke-free laws at the local, state, and regional levels on hospital admissions for heart attacks. To date, all seven published studies of this type have found that smoke-free laws are associated with substantial, rapid reductions in heart attack admissions. Studies of this type are clearly very important, and have major implications for public health practice. However, because these studies involve complex analytical approaches and assess health outcomes in the general population, and not simply among employees of hospitality venues, they are beyond the scope of this publication. Finally, some studies examine the impact of smoke-free laws on smoking behavior. These studies examine several outcomes, including smoking prevalence, quit attempts, successful cessation, and cigarette consumption among continuing smokers. Most of these studies focus on adults, and many focus on the impact of workplace smoking restrictions on employee smoking behavior. While these studies assess an important effect of a smoke-free law, changes in smoking behavior represent a secondary benefit of a smoke-free law and are driven by a number of factors. As a result, these studies are not considered here.

It is never too early or too late to assess the impact of a smoke-free law. Useful studies can be conducted at every stage of the policy process. However, whenever possible, data should be collected before a law takes effect to provide the baseline needed to measure change. If baseline data are unavailable, alternative study designs are necessary (e.g., comparing sites or venues that are and are not covered by the law). These designs generate useful findings, though the findings can be weaker and more open to criticism. Table 1 presents the activities that can be carried out under the five major study domains at each stage in the policy process.

Table 1. Timing of an Evaluation Plan for Smoke-Free Policies

Study	Before the Law Is Passed or Takes Effect	Within One Year of Implementation	One Year or Longer after Implementation
Public support	Assess support.	Assess support.	Assess support.
Compliance	Conduct baseline observations of smoking in hospitality venues.	Assess short-term compliance.	Assess long-term compliance.
Air quality monitoring	Measure baseline air quality in hospitality venues.	Measure short-term changes in air quality.	Measure long-term changes in air quality.
Employee health	Assess baseline worker secondhand smoke exposure and related health effects.	Assess short-term changes in worker secondhand smoke exposure and related health effects.	Assess long-term changes in worker secondhand smoke exposure and related health effects.
Economic impact	Identify available data sources and plan analyses.	As employment data become available, assess the law's impact on hospitality venues.	As taxable sales revenue data become available, assess the law's impact on hospitality venues.

Key Questions to Consider in Choosing Among Study Types

When deciding on an evaluation plan, consider the following questions:

- What stage has the site reached in the policy process? Is the law still under consideration, or has it been enacted? If it has been enacted, has it taken effect? How long has the law been in effect?

- What kinds of information are decision makers, the news media, the business community, and the public requesting? What aspects of the law and its impact are generating the most discussion?

- Does the law contain exemptions or other provisions that have the potential to significantly reduce its reach and impact?

- What resources are available to design and conduct an evaluation?

What stage has the site reached in the policy process? Is the law still under consideration, or has it been enacted? If it has been enacted, has it taken effect? How long has the law been in effect?

If the smoke-free law is under consideration, three types of studies are particularly helpful. Studies to assess public support for the law help determine whether support is strong enough to move ahead with an effort to put a law in place or whether additional public education is necessary. Air quality and employee health studies document air quality in venues that allow smoking and assess secondhand smoke exposure and any related health problems among nonsmoking workers. In addition to these three types of studies, a summary of economic impact studies from sites that have implemented smoke-free laws can provide policy makers with information to address concerns that the law could have a negative economic impact on the local hospitality industry.

Whenever possible, data should be collected before a smoke-free law takes effect in order to establish a baseline. Ideally, data should be collected within 3 months before the law's effective date, within 3 months after this date, and again about 12 months after this date. Collecting data at these intervals may require modifying or supplementing an existing survey, such as the Adult Tobacco Survey (ATS).

During the first year or so after a smoke-free law is implemented, policy makers, the news media, the business community, and the general public are especially interested in the law's effects. Consequently, it is important to be able to report findings on how implementation is proceeding, on whether air quality and employee secondhand smoke exposure in hospitality venues have changed, and on whether the law is having an economic impact on these venues. For example, follow-up assessments of public support conducted shortly after the law takes effect and periodically thereafter can document changes in public support for the law. Similarly, conducting an observational compliance study along with a smaller air quality study in a subset of the same hospitality venues can assess compliance with the law and changes in air quality in these venues. A compliance study can also identify types of venues and regions where intensified educational and enforcement efforts are needed. Finally, although objective local data on the economic impact of the law take longer to become available, it is important to provide policy makers with these data as soon as possible.

In most cases, collecting additional data in all five study domains becomes less critical after a smoke-free law has been in effect for a year. However, in situations where a law has long phase-in provisions for certain venues (e.g., bars or casinos), or where certain venues have been permanently exempted from the law, repeated measurements over longer periods may be needed to document smoking levels, air quality, and employee health in these venues.

What kinds of information are decision makers, the news media, the business community, and the public requesting? What aspects of the law and its impact are generating the most discussion?

Sites should choose studies that address the issues that are generating the most discussion. The following concerns are frequently raised:

- Is there public support for a comprehensive smoke-free law that covers all workplaces and public places, including restaurants and bars?

- Will hospitality venues and smokers comply with the law? Will enforcement be expensive and time-consuming, and will it divert resources from more urgent law enforcement needs?

- Is the air quality in hospitality venues that allow smoking unhealthy? Does the air quality improve following the implementation of a smoke-free law? How effective is installing an advanced ventilation system or creating a separately ventilated smoking room as an alternative to going smoke-free?

- To what extent are nonsmoking restaurant and bar employees exposed to secondhand smoke at work? Is this exposure harmful to employees' health? How do employee exposure on the job and related health outcomes change following the implementation of a smoke-free law?

- Will a smoke-free law have a negative economic impact on restaurants and bars?

Occasionally, it will be necessary to provide local data quickly to policy makers or the media. Public opinion surveys, air quality studies, and observational studies of smoking levels and compliance in hospitality venues can be performed quickly and with fewer resources. Because employee health studies are complex, they cannot be fielded quickly or inexpensively. Economic impact studies cannot be conducted in the immediate post-implementation period because economic data are usually not available for several months after the period in question. If the main questions raised concern employee health or economic impact, the best short-term approach is to summarize the evidence from peer-reviewed studies conducted in other sites that have implemented smoke-free laws and then to make the case that the site in question can expect similar results.

Does the law contain exemptions or other provisions that have the potential to significantly reduce its reach and impact?

Although states and communities are increasingly enacting comprehensive smoke-free laws that contain few exemptions, some smoke-free laws have limitations that need to be taken into account when planning an evaluation. For example, laws may exempt certain types of venues, such as stand-alone bars, private clubs, or casinos, or they may allow smoking in separately ventilated rooms or in adults-only establishments. Laws can include hardship exemptions and waiver provisions that temporarily exempt hospitality venues that can show that the law has hurt their business. Finally, there may be long lag times between the date a law is passed and the date it takes effect in all or certain venues. In these cases, an effective strategy is to design an evaluation to examine the impact these limitations have on a law's effectiveness (e.g., by assessing air quality and employee health in exempted or phased-in hospitality venues, or by examining the impact of exemptions or other provisions on compliance).

What resources are available to design and conduct an evaluation?

Before deciding which studies to pursue, it is important to assess the available resources. Although all studies benefit from careful planning and as much lead time as possible, some studies can be conducted relatively quickly with fewer resources. For example, an observational compliance study that uses volunteer observers can be conducted on a tight time line with limited resources. Other studies are complex and should not be attempted without in-depth planning, substantial lead time, and statistical expertise. These include employee health and economic impact studies. Employee health studies also typically require significant funding.

Additionally, because both public support and employee health studies involve surveying human subjects, and because some employee health studies also involve taking biological specimens or conducting physical exams, these studies may require approval by an Institutional Review Board (IRB). Requirements for IRB review and approval vary by organization. It is important to know and follow the applicable requirements for the organization in question. If IRB approval is required, it is necessary to allow substantial lead time, and it is advisable to consult with a researcher or other resource person who has IRB experience. Lastly, sites should check whether Health Insurance Portability and Accountability Act (HIPAA) regulations apply, especially for employee health studies.

When selecting studies to pursue, consider the following questions about available resources and organizational capacity:

- How much funding is available?

- Is statistical expertise available for survey design and data analysis?

- Are paid staff or volunteers available?

- What data are available or can be obtained?

An additional question to consider is at what level the study will be conducted. If a state smoke-free law is being evaluated, use statewide data. For local laws, use the appropriate level of local data (e.g., city level data for municipal laws, county level data for county laws). The availability of data dictates the type of study that can be conducted. A number of local data sources may be available. For example, for tobacco use behaviors and attitudes, it may be possible to develop sub-state estimates using data collected by the state ATS or the state Behavioral Risk Factor Surveillance System (BRFSS) (see http://apps.nccd.cdc.gov/brfss-smart/index.asp for information on available local BRFSS data by state). As another example, state bureaus of labor statistics can often provide county-level employment data.

EVALUATING THE IMPACT OF SMOKE-FREE POLICIES: OVERVIEW OF AVAILABLE APPROACHES

Section 1 outlines factors to consider when developing an evaluation plan. This section provides in-depth information on the five main types of studies commonly used to evaluate smoke-free laws. It describes the information each study yields, the way this information can be used, the potential pitfalls associated with each study, the optimal times to collect data, and some recommended approaches to use. Table 2 summarizes this information for all five studies.

Public Support

Why Do I Need This Information?

Before the Law Is Passed

The study findings document levels of public awareness of the health effects of secondhand smoke and of the proposed policy and public support for smoke-free environments and for a smoke-free law. Findings can help determine whether support is strong enough to move forward, or if more public education is needed. In addition, the findings establish a baseline to measure change.

After the Law Is Implemented

The study findings document levels of public support and changes in these levels over time. These findings help document shifts in social norms by tracking trends in support for the law and for smoke-free environments in specific types of venues.

What Information Will I Get?

The study findings document the proportion of the public that supports the law and how this support changes over time. Findings can also be used to determine the support for extending the law to cover venues exempted permanently or for phase-in periods. In addition, it may be possible to assess public awareness and concern regarding the health effects of secondhand smoke and changes in these beliefs and attitudes that may occur because of the discussion regarding and the implementation of the smoke-free law and related media coverage or paid media campaigns.

What Pitfalls Should I Guard Against?

Because the study involves human subjects, check the relevant institution's IRB requirements. When developing survey questions, choose unbiased wording to safeguard the validity and credibility of the study and its findings. Using standard questions from existing surveys or publicly available questionnaires is useful to allow the study results to be compared to other studies with the same questions. A helpful source of standard survey questions is the CDC Office on Smoking and Health's Question Inventory on Tobacco (http://apps.nccd.cdc.gov/QIT/QuickSearch.aspx).

When Do I Need This Information?

Collecting pre-implementation data is important to assess public readiness, to document levels of public support, and to establish a baseline to measure change. Collecting post-implementation data helps track changes in public support and shifts in social norms over time. If possible, data should be collected within 3 months before the law takes effect, within 3 months after this date, and at regular intervals thereafter (e.g., annually). This may require innovative approaches such as conducting rolling quarterly surveys or special surveys.

Possible Approaches

One approach to assess public attitudes is to analyze data from existing population health surveys, such as the Adult Tobacco Survey (ATS) (in states that conduct this survey) or the Behavioral Risk Factor Surveillance System (BRFSS), that already include relevant questions. If such a survey lacks relevant questions, a second approach is to add those questions to the survey. A third approach is to conduct a public opinion survey using a probability sample. Keep in mind that this approach is substantially more expensive than the other options. Each of these approaches requires expertise in survey administration and analysis and may involve obtaining IRB approval.

Compliance

Why Do I Need This Information?

The enactment of a smoke-free law does not automatically result in smoke-free workplaces and public places. For a law to reduce secondhand smoke exposure, compliance levels must be high. Observational compliance studies assess whether this is the case. In addition to documenting compliance levels and monitoring trends in compliance over time, these studies can identify specific types of venues or regions where increased educational and enforcement efforts are needed. In sites where adequate planning and extensive communication with business owners and the public have occurred, observational compliance studies typically find that most workplaces and businesses, including most hospitality venues, come into compliance with a law shortly after it takes effect.

What Information Will I Get?

This study provides data on the proportion of hospitality venues that are complying with the law. Compliance is assessed by observing the smoking levels in these venues and the measures that these venues take to comply, such as posting "No Smoking" signs and removing ashtrays. Compliance can also be assessed by determining the proportion of patrons who report that they observed smoking the last time they visited a restaurant or bar.

By collecting pre- and post-implementation data, it is possible to document whether the proportion of hospitality venues where smoking occurs changes after the law takes effect. Conducting assessments at two or more intervals following implementation allows sites to monitor trends in compliance over time. (Because the law is not yet in effect, baseline data measure the presence of smoking in hospitality venues, not compliance.)

What Pitfalls Should I Guard Against?

Be prepared to encounter less than full compliance. Certain types of venues and geographic areas (e.g., bars, rural areas, communities that lack previous experience with local smoke-free laws) often take longer than others to achieve high compliance rates. A compliance study can indicate types of venues and areas that could benefit from intensified educational and enforcement efforts. Plan to conduct observations during peak business hours to ensure that the results reflect real-world conditions.

When Do I Need This Information?

Ideally, compliance data should be collected within 3 months before the law takes effect, within 3 months afterward, and thereafter at regular intervals, such as annually, if possible. This may require innovative approaches such as rolling quarterly surveys or special surveys. Pre-implementation data are not essential, but are highly recommended as a baseline to assess change. Data collected soon after the law takes effect help document short-term compliance levels and inform education and enforcement activities. Longer-term data help document ongoing compliance levels, track trends in compliance, and inform education and enforcement activities.

Possible Approaches

The most cost-effective approach to assess compliance is to draw on an existing population health survey, such as a state ATS or BRFSS, that already includes relevant questions. Another fairly inexpensive approach is to add relevant questions to such a survey. A third approach is to conduct an observational study, which can be relatively inexpensive if it makes use of volunteers from partner organizations.

A fourth approach is to analyze enforcement agency records on complaints, violations, and citations. This approach should be used to complement other approaches, not as the sole source of data, because these data do not reflect all the violations of the law and can be difficult to interpret. For example, a small number of citations can reflect either high compliance or lack of enforcement. Similarly, an increase in citations can reflect either a decrease in compliance or an increase in enforcement, and an increase in complaints can reflect either decreased compliance or increased publicity about the law. However, because the level of enforcement influences the interpretation of enforcement agency records and is an important determinant of compliance with a smoke-free law, evaluations of compliance should assess and take account of enforcement activities.

Air Quality Monitoring

Why Do I Need This Information?

Before the Law Is Passed

These studies document air quality in restaurants, bars, and other hospitality venues that allow smoking. Pre-implementation data are essential for establishing a baseline to measure change.

After the Law Is Implemented

Measurements taken before and after a smoke-free law takes effect document changes in air quality. Air quality studies can be conducted relatively quickly and can provide real-time data.

What Information Will I Get?

It will be possible to collect information on the concentrations of respirable suspended particles or particulate matter present in hospitality venues, which are measures of air quality. The data collected will also include the cigarette density (average number of burning cigarettes) in a venue, the average number of persons present, the volume of the venue, and the presence of signs about the venue's smoking policy.

What Pitfalls Should I Guard Against?

This study requires sites to purchase, rent, or borrow air quality monitoring equipment and related computer software and to train data collectors to use the equipment. In addition, measurements should be taken during peak business hours to reflect real-world conditions. Lastly, to ensure that data processing and analysis are performed correctly, it is best to have researchers supervise these steps.

When Do I Need This Information?

Ideally, air quality data should be collected within 3 months before and within 3 months after the law takes effect. Baseline data are very important for this type of study. Pre-implementation data are needed to assess post-implementation changes in air quality in venues. An additional wave of data collection (e.g., 1 year after the law's effective date) may be useful, but is not necessary.

Possible Approaches

The necessary equipment and software are not prohibitively expensive. Monitoring can be carried out either by volunteers or by professional data collectors, though all data collectors must be trained prior to conducting measurements. An air quality study can be conducted in conjunction with a compliance study by taking air quality measurements in a subset of the venues visited during the compliance study.

Employee Health

Why Do I Need This Information?

Before the Law Is Passed

This information documents secondhand smoke exposure and related health effects among nonsmoking employees in hospitality venues that allow smoking. Collecting pre-implementation data is essential to assess changes in employee exposure and health outcomes following implementation of the law.

After the Law Is Implemented

Reduced secondhand smoke exposure and improved health outcomes among nonsmoking hospitality workers after a law is implemented can help demonstrate that the law is achieving its purpose. Conversely, persistent or increasing secondhand smoke exposure and health problems among workers in hospitality venues exempt from the law can demonstrate the benefit of extending protections to these workers.

What Information Will I Get?

These studies provide both objective and self-reported data on changes in secondhand smoke exposure and health outcomes among nonsmoking employees in hospitality venues. A common objective measure is the level of cotinine, a metabolite of nicotine which is used as a biomarker of secondhand smoke exposure. Cotinine can be measured in saliva, urine, or blood. Saliva measurements are least expensive and least intrusive. Detectable cotinine levels indicate that nonsmoking workers are exposed to secondhand smoke, and higher cotinine levels indicate higher levels of exposure. Another objective measure is the level of NNAL, a marker for exposure to the tobacco-specific lung carcinogen NNK. NNAL is typically measured in urine, generally in conjunction with measurements of cotinine. Detectable levels of NNAL demonstrate the presence of a potent carcinogen in the bodies of employees who have been exposed to secondhand smoke in the workplace. This is an intermediate step toward demonstrating that secondhand smoke exposure is causing health effects in workers. A third objective measure is to use spirometry to assess lung function. In addition to assessing objective measures, employee health studies also typically collect self-reported data on secondhand smoke exposure and respiratory and sensory symptoms.

What Pitfalls Should I Guard Against?

Employee health studies are complex and time-intensive and can be expensive. They require considerable planning and adequate lead time to design the study, to recruit participants, and to obtain baseline data before a law takes effect. Depending on an organization's funding source and requirements, IRB approval may be required to conduct interviews, take saliva or urine samples, and perform measurements of lung function.

Additionally, it is best to collaborate with researchers experienced in collecting and analyzing biological samples and, if necessary, in IRB procedures. Lastly, these studies require access to laboratory services to analyze saliva and urine samples for the presence of biomarkers.

When Do I Need This Information?

Baseline data are essential for this study and should be collected within 3 months before the law takes effect. Post-implementation data should be collected within 3 months after the law takes effect to document short-term changes. Another round of data collection one year after the law takes effect is useful to document long-term changes.

Possible Approaches

Employee health studies are typically the most expensive study to conduct because of the need for laboratory and clinical resources and for multiple waves of data collection. Common study designs include (1) self-collected, mailed-in saliva cotinine samples, combined with telephone surveys assessing self-reported secondhand smoke exposure and respiratory and sensory symptoms; (2) clinic-based urine studies measuring cotinine and/or NNAL levels; and (3) spirometry to measure lung function, combined with personal interviews.

The first approach is relatively inexpensive, while the second and third approaches require significant funding. It is important to secure funding, identify research partners, and arrange for access to clinical resources well in advance. If possible, combine measurements of cotinine with measurements of NNAL and combine monitoring of self-reported respiratory symptoms with clinical measurements of lung function.

Economic Impact

Why Do I Need This Information?

Before the Law Is Passed
Objective data from economic impact studies conducted in other sites that have implemented smoke-free laws can be used to address concerns among policy makers and proprietors of hospitality venues about the law's potential economic impact on restaurants and bars.

After the Law Is Implemented
Objective local economic data are useful to gauge the law's aggregate economic impact on all hospitality venues in a jurisdiction. Concerns about a law's impact often peak immediately after the law takes effect and largely subside after a year.

What Information Will I Get?
Economic impact studies focus primarily on hospitality venues, most commonly restaurants and bars, because these are generally the focus of debate. Employment levels and taxable sales revenue are the two types of objective data most often used to gauge economic impact, and are currently the indicators of choice in this area. Other indicators include the number of venues that have opened or closed, hotel revenues and occupancy levels, the number of licenses issued to restaurants and bars, and self-reported consumer patronage intentions and patterns.

What Pitfalls Should I Guard Against?
Policy makers and other groups frequently ask for reports on the economic impact of a law before objective local data are available. It is important to be prepared to respond to policy makers' concerns and to claims that the law is having a negative economic impact on hospitality venues. Reporting on economic impact data can be problematic because of the time it takes for these data to become available. Employment data have the quickest turnaround, but still take 6–9 months after the month in question. Taxable sales revenue data take about 18 months after the quarter in question. In addition, for a study to be considered reliable in determining trends, it will need to include enough data points before and after the law (at least one year of data after the law's effective date), and it will need to control for underlying economic trends and seasonal factors. For example, any analysis of bar employment or sales needs to take into account the fact that the stand-alone bar industry has declined in recent years. Whenever possible, it is best to collaborate with researchers with econometric or statistical expertise, especially when conducting more sophisticated analyses.

When Do I Need This Information?
For this study, collecting baseline data is not necessary because government agencies routinely collect these data. During the policy adoption phase, objective economic data from other sites that have implemented smoke-free laws should be used to respond to policy makers' questions. Once the law is implemented, objective local economic data are needed as soon as possible to address any concerns or claims that the law is adversely impacting hospitality venues.

Possible Approaches

Most economic impact studies involve obtaining and analyzing publicly available data on employment (e.g., Current Employment Statistics [CES] data), taxable sales revenues, business openings and closings, or some combination of these measures. These data are often available either free of charge or for a small processing fee from government agencies. Relevant agencies include state bureaus of labor statistics and state departments of labor, revenue, and taxation and finance.

Another approach is to add a question on consumer patronage intentions or patterns to an existing survey, such as the ATS. However, this information should be used to complement objective data, not as the sole data source. Ideally, an economic impact study should compare economic trends in the site in question to trends in a control site that has not implemented a smoke-free law.

Table 2. Evaluating the Impact of Smoke-Free Policies: Overview of Available Approaches

Type of Study	Why Do I Need This Information?	What Information Will I Get?	What Pitfalls Should I Guard Against?	When Do I Need This Information?	Possible Approaches (Relative Cost: $ to $$$$)
Public Support	Before the law is passed: • To assess public awareness of the health effects of secondhand smoke and of the proposed law. • To assess public readiness. • To document the level of public support for smoke-free environments and for the proposed law. • To establish a baseline for measuring change. After the law is implemented: • To assess levels of public support for the law and changes in these levels over time. • To document shifts in social norms. • To monitor public support for extending the law to cover additional venues.	• The proportion of the population that supports the law and how this changes over time. • The proportion of the population that supports extending the law to additional venues. • The proportion of the population that is aware of and concerned about the health effects of secondhand smoke.	• Institutional Review Board (IRB) approval may be required to conduct surveys. Check on IRB requirements. • Take care to use unbiased wording on survey questions. • If possible, use standard questions from existing, publicly available surveys.	• If possible, data should be collected within 3 months before the law takes effect, within 3 months after this date, and at regular intervals thereafter (e.g., annually).	• Use existing population health surveys, such as the Adult Tobacco Survey (ATS) or the Behavioral Risk Factor Surveillance System (BRFSS), that include relevant questions. • Add questions to an existing population health survey such as the ATS or BRFSS ($). • Conduct your own public opinion survey using a probability sample ($$$–$$$$).
Compliance	After the law is implemented: • To assess compliance with the law.	• The proportion of hospitality venues that comply with the law (i.e., no observed smoking), and how this changes over time.	• Do not expect full compliance in all venues. • Certain types of venues and certain geographic regions often take longer than others to achieve high compliance rates.	• Although not essential, collecting baseline data before the law goes into effect makes it possible to assess changes in smoking levels in hospitality venues.	• Use existing population health surveys, such as the ATS or BRFSS, that include relevant questions. • Add questions to an existing population health survey, such as the ATS or BRFSS ($).

Type of Study	Why Do I Need This Information?	What Information Will I Get?	What Pitfalls Should I Guard Against?	When Do I Need This Information?	Possible Approaches (Relative Cost: $ to $$$$)
Compliance (continued)	• To identify types of venues and geographic regions where increased educational and enforcement efforts are needed. • To monitor compliance over time in order to assess trends and address any new problem areas.	• Information on measures hospitality venues take to comply with the law (e.g., posting "No Smoking" signs, removing ashtrays). • The proportion of patrons who report having observed smoking in venues.	• Conduct observations during peak business hours to reflect real-world conditions.	• If possible, data should be collected within 3 months before the law takes effect, within 3 months afterward, and thereafter at regular intervals (e.g., annually).	• Conduct an observational study using volunteers from partner organizations ($). • Analyze enforcement agency records. (Use to complement other approaches, not as the sole information source.)
Air Quality Monitoring	Before the law is passed: • To document air quality in hospitality venues that allow smoking. • To establish a baseline for measuring change. After the law is implemented: • To document changes in air quality.	• Concentrations of respirable suspended particles or particulate matter. • Cigarette density (average number of burning cigarettes). • Average number of persons present. • The volume of the venue. • Signs about the venue's smoking policy.	• Air quality monitoring equipment and computer software are required. • Data collectors must be trained to use the equipment. • Obtain air quality measurements during peak business hours to reflect real-world conditions. • Data processing and analysis should be supervised by researchers.	• If possible, data should be collected within 3 months before the law takes effect and within 3 months after this date. An additional wave of data collection (e.g., 1 year after the law's effective date) may be useful, but is not essential.	• Equipment and software expenses should be moderate ($–$$). • Volunteers or staff are needed to conduct the measurements. • This study can be carried out in a subset of the hospitality venues included in a larger observational compliance study ($–$$).
Employee Health	Before the law is passed: • To document secondhand smoke exposure and related health problems among nonsmoking workers in hospitality venues that allow smoking. After the law is implemented: • To document changes in secondhand smoke exposure and related health problems among nonsmoking workers in venues covered by the law. • To document exposure and related health problems among workers in hospitality venues not covered by the law, and to compare these outcomes to outcomes for workers in covered venues.	• Levels of cotinine (a biomarker for second-hand smoke exposure) in saliva or urine, and the proportion of workers with cotinine levels above the limit of detection. • Prevalence and duration of self-reported second-hand smoke exposure. • Prevalence of self-reported sensory and respiratory symptoms. • Levels of NNAL (a bio-marker for exposure to the tobacco-specific lung carcinogen NNK) in urine, and the proportion of workers with NNAL levels above the limit of detection. • Clinical measures of lung function (spirometry). • How these indicators change over time after the law takes effect.	• Employee health studies are complicated and time-intensive, and require careful planning and substantial lead time. • IRB approval may be needed to conduct surveys or interviews, to take saliva or urine samples, and to measure lung function. Check on IRB requirements. • If possible, collaborate with researchers experienced in collecting and analyzing biological samples and, if necessary, experienced in IRB procedures. • Laboratory services are needed to analyze saliva or urine samples. • Recruiting participants can be time-consuming and costly.	• Baseline data should be collected within 3 months before the law takes effect. • Follow-up data from the same workers sampled at baseline should be collected within 3 months after the law takes effect to document its short-term effects. • It is helpful to collect data again 1 year after the law takes effect to document long-term changes in employee exposure and health effects.	• A study using self-collected, mailed-in saliva cotinine specimens combined with a telephone survey assessing self-reported secondhand smoke exposure and sensory and respiratory symptoms in nonsmoking hospitality workers ($$$). • A study of cotinine levels and, if possible, NNAL levels in urine, combined with personal interviews ($$$). • Measurement of lung function using spirometry, combined with personal interviews ($$$).

Type of Study	Why Do I Need This Information?	What Information Will I Get?	What Pitfalls Should I Guard Against?	When Do I Need This Information?	Possible Approaches (Relative Cost: $ to $$$$)
Economic Impact	Before the law is passed: • Findings from objective economic impact studies conducted in other sites with smoke-free laws can address stakeholder concerns about the law's potential impact on hospitality venues. After the law is implemented: • Objective local economic data provide information about the law's economic impact on hospitality venues.	Information on the economic impact of the law on hospitality venues, including: • Employment levels, which are typically available in monthly increments, often from Current Employment Statistics (CES) data. • Taxable sales revenue, which is typically available in quarterly increments. • The number of venues that have opened or closed. • The number of licenses issued to restaurants and bars. • Self-reported consumer patronage intentions or patterns.	• Anticipate high interest among policy makers, who may request reports on a law's economic impact before objective information is available. • It takes time for objective economic data to become available: about 6–9 months for employment data and about 18 months for taxable sales revenue data. • Have enough data points before and after the law to determine trends reliably (at least one year of data after the law's effective date). • Control for underlying economic trends and seasonal variations. • Econometric or statistical expertise is necessary to conduct more sophisticated analyses.	• Before the law is passed, use findings of objective studies conducted in other smoke-free sites to address decision makers' concerns. • After the law takes effect, analyze objective economic data as this information becomes available and report findings. • Baseline data do not need to be collected before the law takes effect; these data are routinely collected by government agencies and should be available later.	• Obtain and analyze publicly available data on employment levels, taxable sales revenue, business openings and closings, and licenses issued. These data should be available free or for a nominal fee from appropriate government agencies (e.g., state departments of revenue, state departments of taxation and finance, state departments of labor, state bureaus of labor statistics). • Add a question on consumer patronage intentions or patterns to an existing survey, such as the ATS. (Use to complement other approaches, not as the sole information source.) ($) • If possible, in addition to comparing economic indicators in your site before and after the law takes effect, compare data from your site to data from a similar control site that has not implemented a smoke-free law.

STEP-BY-STEP GUIDE TO SELECTING APPROPRIATE EVALUATION STUDIES FOR SMOKE-FREE POLICIES

This section is primarily intended for use by public health professionals who are providing technical assistance to state or local tobacco control programs to help these programs plan how to evaluate a proposed or existing state or local smoke-free law. The steps presented in this section help to identify appropriate studies to conduct on the basis of four factors:

1. The stage the site has reached in the policy process.

2. The key issues that have emerged in the policy debate and that are of greatest interest to policy makers, other community leaders, the news media, the business community, and the public.

3. Any major exemptions in the smoke-free law.

4. The level of resources available.

These factors help programs select studies that are feasible and that provide the information necessary for an evaluation.

Key Questions

The person providing technical assistance can quickly assess the situation by asking the following four questions:

1. What stage has the site reached in the policy process?

   - The law has not yet been passed.

   - The law has been passed but not implemented.

   - The law has been in effect for less than 1 year.

   - The law has been in effect for 1 year or longer.

2. What are the key issues?

   - Public support for the law.

   - Compliance with the law.

   - Air quality and secondhand smoke levels in hospitality venues.

   - Secondhand smoke exposure and related health effects among nonsmoking employees of hospitality venues.

   - The economic impact of the law on hospitality venues.

3. Does the proposed or existing law contain major exemptions? These can include the following:

- Exemptions for bars, restaurant bar areas, casinos, bingo venues, other gaming venues, bowling alleys, billiard parlors, private clubs, or other specific venues.

- Ventilation provisions.

- Provisions allowing smoking in adults-only settings.

- Economic hardship exemptions.

- Long phase-in periods (longer than 3 months) for certain settings, such as bars and casinos.

- Other provisions that create gaps in coverage or weaken protections.

4. What resources are available?

- Funding: minimal, moderate (<$25,000), or significant (≥$25,000).

- Labor (including paid staff and volunteers).

- Access to an Institutional Review Board (IRB).

- Access to statistical expertise for survey design, implementation, and data analysis.

Study Recommendations

Before the Policy is Passed or Implemented

Useful studies to conduct during this phase include assessing public support for a smoke-free law, observing the level of smoking in hospitality venues, measuring air quality in these venues, and assessing secondhand smoke exposure and related health effects among nonsmoking workers in these venues. It is also helpful to begin identifying data sources to use for economic impact studies.

Whenever possible, sites should collect baseline data before the law takes effect. The combination of baseline data and data collected after the law has taken effect is essential for showing that changes occurred in key outcomes after the law was implemented. To be comparable, all data must be collected using the same methods. Collecting baseline data is especially critical for employee health studies and is important for air quality and compliance studies as well. Although public support studies benefit from baseline data, in this case these data are not crucial. If sites are unable to collect data before the law is passed, they can still do so in the interim between when the law is passed and when it takes effect.

Sites need to consider the level of resources available (i.e., minimal, moderate, or significant) both when selecting among the five broad study types and when selecting the specific approach to use in conducting each type of study.

In this section, we use the terms "probability sample" and "convenience sample" to describe two different ways to generate a sample of people or venues for a study. A probability sample is a true probabilistic, or random, sample designed by a specialist in statistical survey methodology. This method is preferred whenever an organization has the resources to take this approach. A convenience sample is not a true probability sample. This approach is used primarily when sampling venues for compliance or for air quality.

A convenience sample of venues is typically small, with fewer than 20 venues, and it deliberately includes all of the main types of venues present in the study site. The goal of a convenience sample is to choose a sample of venues that is "representative" of the venues in the study site without the burden of designing a probability sample. This approach should be adopted only by sites that lack the resources to select a true probability sample.

Sites should select the specific approach they take in conducting each type of study on the basis of their level of resources.

Minimal Resources: small community partner (no funding, no paid staff, volunteers only).

- **Public Support**

    Use an existing population health survey, such as the Adult Tobacco Survey (ATS), that includes relevant questions.

- **Compliance**

    ■ Use an existing population health survey that includes relevant questions.

    ■ Have volunteers conduct observations in a convenience sample of hospitality venues.

- **Air Quality Monitoring**

    Rent or borrow an air quality monitoring device and have volunteers collect data in a convenience sample of hospitality venues.

- **Employee Health**

    ■ An original study is not feasible.

    ■ Summarize findings of peer-reviewed studies from other smoke-free sites and make the case that similar results can be expected in your community.

- **Economic Impact**

    ■ An original study is not feasible.

    ■ Summarize findings of peer-reviewed studies from other smoke-free sites and make the case that similar results can be expected in your community.

Moderate Resources: organized community coalition, small health department (limited or significant funding, paid staff, access to many volunteers).

- **Public Support**

  - Use an existing population health survey that includes relevant questions.

  - Pay to add one or more questions to an existing population health survey.

- **Compliance**

  - Use an existing population health survey that includes relevant questions.

  - Pay to add one or more questions to an existing population health survey.

  - Have volunteers conduct observations in a convenience sample of hospitality venues.

- **Air Quality Monitoring**

  Purchase, rent, or borrow an air quality monitoring device and have volunteers collect data in a convenience sample of hospitality venues.

- **Employee Health**

  - An original study is not feasible.

  - Summarize findings of peer-reviewed studies from other smoke-free sites and make the case that similar results can be expected in your community.

- **Economic Impact**

  - Pay an economic or statistical consultant to collect and analyze economic data.

  - Summarize findings of peer-reviewed studies from other smoke-free sites and make the case that similar results can be expected in your community.

  - Lack of baseline data is not an issue with economic data, because historical data are typically available from government agencies.

Significant Resources: large community partners, state health department, involvement of other partners, such as voluntary organizations, national organizations, funders, or researchers (significant funding, large paid staff, large network of volunteers, access to IRB, statistical expertise, and laboratory services).

- **Public Support**

  Conduct a population survey using a probability sample.

- **Compliance**

  - Have volunteers conduct observations in a convenience or probability sample of hospitality venues.

  - Use an existing population health survey that includes relevant questions, or add one or more questions to such a survey.

- **Air Quality Monitoring**

  Purchase one or more air quality monitoring devices and have volunteers, contractors, or environmental health staff collect data in a convenience or probability sample of hospitality venues.

- **Employee Health**

    - ■ Conduct a study using self-collected and mailed-in saliva cotinine specimens from nonsmoking workers in hospitality venues, combined with a telephone survey assessing self-reported secondhand smoke exposure and respiratory and sensory symptoms among these workers.

    - ■ If more funding is available, conduct a study measuring NNAL in urine and/or measuring lung function using spirometry, combined with personal interviews, among nonsmoking hospitality workers.

    - ■ Baseline data are essential.

- **Economic Impact**

    - ■ Collect and analyze relevant economic data.

    - ■ Lack of baseline data is not an issue with economic data, because historical data are typically available from government agencies.

Within One Year of Implementation

Useful studies to conduct during this phase include assessing public support for the smoke-free law, assessing compliance, measuring air quality in hospitality venues, and assessing secondhand smoke exposure and related health effects among nonsmoking hospitality employees. Because of the long lag times in the availability of economic data, the first economic impact studies (which rely on employment data) must typically wait until 6–9 months after the law takes effect. Some studies can be conducted in a way that partially compensates for a lack of baseline data.

Sites should select the specific approach they take in conducting each type of study on the basis of their level of resources.

Minimal Resources: small community partner (no funding, no paid staff, volunteers only).

- **Public Support**

    - ■ Use an existing population health survey that includes relevant questions.

    - ■ Although baseline data are optimal, they are not essential. Check whether existing state population health surveys have relevant historical data.

- **Compliance**

    - ■ Use an existing population health survey that includes relevant questions.

    - ■ Have volunteers conduct observations in a convenience sample of hospitality venues.

    - ■ If baseline data are unavailable, consider collecting and comparing data on smoking levels in hospitality venues from jurisdictions or venues not subject to the proposed law.

- **Air Quality Monitoring**

    - ■ Rent or borrow an air quality monitoring device and have volunteers collect data in a convenience sample of hospitality venues.

    - ■ If baseline data are unavailable, consider collecting and comparing data from jurisdictions or venues not subject to the proposed law.

- **Employee Health**

  - ■ An original study is not feasible.

  - ■ Summarize findings of peer-reviewed studies from other smoke-free sites and make the case that similar results can be expected in your community.

- **Economic Impact**

  - ■ An original study is not feasible.

  - ■ Summarize findings of peer-reviewed studies from other smoke-free sites and make the case that similar results can be expected in your community.

Moderate Resources: organized community coalition, small health department (limited or significant funding, paid staff, access to many volunteers).

- **Public Support**

  - ■ Use an existing population health survey that includes relevant questions.

  - ■ Pay to add one or more questions to an existing population health survey.

  - ■ Although baseline data are optimal, they are not essential. Check whether existing state population health surveys have relevant historical data.

- **Compliance**

  - ■ Use an existing population health survey that includes relevant questions.

  - ■ Pay to add one or more questions to an existing population health survey.

  - ■ Have volunteers conduct observations in a convenience sample of hospitality venues.

  - ■ If baseline data are unavailable, consider collecting and comparing data from jurisdictions or venues not subject to the proposed law.

- **Air Quality Monitoring**

  - ■ Purchase, rent, or borrow an air quality monitoring device and have volunteers collect data in a convenience sample of hospitality venues.

  - ■ If baseline data are unavailable, consider collecting and comparing data from jurisdictions or venues not subject to the proposed law.

- **Employee Health**

  - ■ An original study is not feasible.

  - ■ Summarize findings of peer-reviewed studies from other smoke-free sites and make the case that similar results can be expected in your community.

- **Economic Impact**

  - ■ Pay an economic or statistical consultant to collect and analyze economic data.

  - ■ Summarize findings of peer-reviewed studies from other smoke-free sites and make the case that similar results can be expected in your community.

  - ■ Lack of baseline data is not an issue with economic data, because historical data are typically available from government agencies.

Significant Resources: large community partners, state health department, involvement of other partners, such as voluntary organizations, national organizations, funders, or researchers (significant funding, large paid staff, large network of volunteers, access to IRB, statistical expertise, and laboratory services).

- **Public Support**
    - ■ Conduct a population survey using a probability sample.
    - ■ Although baseline data are optimal, they are not essential. Check whether existing state population health surveys have relevant historical data.

- **Compliance**
    - ■ Have volunteers conduct observations in a convenience or probability sample of hospitality venues.
    - ■ Use an existing population health survey that includes relevant questions, or add one or more questions to such a survey.
    - ■ If baseline data are unavailable, consider collecting and comparing data from jurisdictions or venues not subject to the proposed law.

- **Air Quality Monitoring**
    - ■ Purchase one or more air quality monitoring devices and have volunteers, contractors, or environmental health staff collect data in a convenience or probability sample of hospitality venues.
    - ■ If baseline data are unavailable, consider collecting and comparing data from jurisdictions or venues not subject to the proposed law.

- **Employee Health**
    - ■ Conduct a study using self-collected and mailed-in saliva cotinine specimens from nonsmoking workers in hospitality venues, combined with a telephone survey assessing self-reported secondhand smoke exposure and respiratory and sensory symptoms among these workers.
    - ■ If more funding is available, conduct a study measuring NNAL in urine and/or measuring lung function using spirometry, combined with personal interviews, among nonsmoking hospitality workers.
    - ■ Baseline data are essential.

- **Economic Impact**
    - ■ Collect and analyze relevant economic data.
    - ■ Lack of baseline data is not an issue with economic data, because historical data are typically available from government agencies.

One Year or Longer After Implementation

Useful studies to conduct during this phase include assessing long-term public support for the smoke-free law, assessing compliance, measuring air quality in hospitality venues, assessing secondhand smoke exposure and related health effects among nonsmoking hospitality workers, and assessing economic impact on hospitality venues by measuring employment levels and taxable sales revenue. Some studies can be conducted in a way that partially compensates for a lack of baseline data.

Sites should select the specific approach they take in conducting each type of study on the basis of their level of resources.

Minimal Resources: small community partner (no funding, no paid staff, volunteers only).

- **Public Support**
    - Use an existing population health survey that includes relevant questions.
    - Although baseline data are optimal, they are not essential. Check whether existing state population health surveys have relevant historical data.

- **Compliance**
    - Use an existing population health survey that includes relevant questions.
    - Have volunteers conduct observations in a convenience sample of hospitality venues.
    - If baseline data are unavailable, consider collecting and comparing data from jurisdictions or venues not subject to the proposed law.

- **Air Quality Monitoring**
    - Rent or borrow an air quality monitoring device and have volunteers collect data in a convenience sample of hospitality venues.
    - If baseline data are unavailable, consider collecting and comparing data from jurisdictions or venues not subject to the proposed law.

- **Employee Health**
    - An original study is not feasible.
    - Summarize findings of peer-reviewed studies from other smoke-free sites and make the case that similar results can be expected in your community.

- **Economic Impact**
    - An original study is not feasible.
    - Summarize findings of peer-reviewed studies from other smoke-free sites and make the case that similar results can be expected in your community.

Moderate Resources: organized community coalition, small health department (limited or significant funding, paid staff, access to many volunteers).

- **Public Support**

    - Use an existing population health survey that includes relevant questions.

    - Pay to add a question to an existing population health survey.

    - Although baseline data are optimal, they are not essential. Check whether existing state population health surveys have relevant historical data.

- **Compliance**

    - Use an existing population health survey that includes relevant questions.

    - Pay to add a question to an existing population health survey.

    - Have volunteers conduct observations in a convenience sample of hospitality venues.

    - If baseline data are unavailable, consider collecting and comparing data from jurisdictions or venues not subject to the proposed law.

- **Air Quality Monitoring**

    - Purchase, rent, or borrow an air quality monitoring device and have volunteers collect data in a convenience sample of hospitality venues.

    - If baseline data are unavailable, consider collecting and comparing data from jurisdictions or venues not subject to the proposed law.

- **Employee Health**

    - An original study is not feasible.

    - Summarize findings of peer-reviewed studies from other smoke-free sites and make the case that similar results can be expected in your community.

- **Economic Impact**

    - Pay an economic or statistical consultant to collect and analyze economic data.

    - Summarize findings of peer-reviewed studies from other smoke-free sites and make the case that similar results can be expected in your community.

    - Lack of baseline data is not an issue with economic data, because historical data are typically available from government agencies.

Significant Resources: large community partners, state health department, involvement of other partners, such as voluntary organizations, national organizations, funders, or researchers (significant funding, large paid staff, large network of volunteers, access to IRB, statistical expertise, and laboratory services).

- **Public Support**

    - Conduct a population survey using a probability sample.

    - Although baseline data are optimal, they are not essential. Check whether existing state population health surveys have relevant historical data.

- **Compliance**

  - ■ Have volunteers conduct observations in a convenience or probability sample of hospitality venues.

  - ■ Use an existing population health survey that includes relevant questions, or add one or more questions to such a survey.

  - ■ If baseline data are unavailable, consider collecting and comparing data from jurisdictions or venues not subject to the proposed law.

- **Air Quality Monitoring**

  - ■ Purchase one or more air quality monitoring devices and have volunteers, contractors, or environmental health staff collect data in a convenience or probability sample of hospitality venues.

  - ■ If baseline data are unavailable, consider collecting and comparing data from jurisdictions or venues not subject to the proposed law.

- **Employee Health**

  - ■ Conduct a study using self-collected and mailed-in saliva cotinine specimens from nonsmoking workers in hospitality venues, combined with a telephone survey assessing self-reported secondhand smoke exposure and respiratory and sensory symptoms among these workers.

  - ■ If more funding is available, conduct a study measuring NNAL in urine and/or measuring lung function using spirometry, combined with personal interviews, among nonsmoking hospitality workers.

  - ■ Baseline data are essential.

- **Economic Impact**

  - ■ Collect and analyze relevant economic data.

  - ■ Lack of baseline data is not an issue with economic data, because historical data are typically available from government agencies.

SELECTED BIBLIOGRAPHY

The following bibliography includes published studies under each of the five domains addressed in this publication. These citations are provided as examples of methodologically sound studies, rather than as a comprehensive listing of studies that have been conducted in these areas.

Public Support

Tang H, Cowling DW, Lloyd JC, Rogers T, Koumjian KL, Stevens CM, Bal DG. Changes of attitudes and patronage behaviors in response to a smoke-free bar law. Am J Public Health 2003;93(4):611–617.

Tang H, Cowling DW, Stevens CM, Lloyd JC. Changes of knowledge, attitudes, beliefs, and preference of bar owner and staff in response to a smoke-free bar law. Tob Control 2004;13(1):87–89.

Compliance

Hyland A, Cummings KM, Wilson MP. Compliance with the New York City Smoke-Free Air Act. J Public Health Manag Prac 1999;5(1):43–52.

Tang H, Cowling DW, Lloyd JC, Rogers T, Koumjian KL, Stevens CM, Bal DG. Changes of attitudes and patronage behaviors in response to a smoke-free bar law. Am J Public Health 2003;93(4):611–617.

Tang H, Cowling DW, Stevens CM, Lloyd JC. Changes of knowledge, attitudes, beliefs, and preference of bar owner and staff in response to a smoke-free bar law. Tob Control 2004;13(1):87–89.

Weber MD, Bagwell DAS, Fielding JE, Glantz SA. Long term compliance with California's Smoke-Free Workplace Law among bars and restaurants in Los Angeles County. Tob Control 2003;12(3):269–273.

Air Quality Monitoring

Centers for Disease Control and Prevention. Indoor air quality in hospitality venues before and after implementation of a clean indoor air law—Western New York, 2003. MMWR 2004;53(44):1038–1041. A

Repace J. Respirable particles and carcinogens in the air of Delaware hospitality venues before and after a smoking ban. J Occup Environ Med 2004;46(9):887–905.

Employee Health

Eisner MD, Smith AK, Blanc PD. Bartenders' respiratory health after establishment of smoke-free bars and taverns. JAMA 1998;280(22):1909–1914. A

Farrelly MC, Nonnemaker JM, Chou R, Hyland A, Peterson KK, Bauer UE. Changes in hospitality workers' exposure to secondhand smoke following the implementation of New York's smoke-free law. Tob Control 2005;14(4):236–241.

Menzies D, Nair A, Williamson PA, Schembri S, Al-Khairalla MZH, Barnes M, et al. Respiratory symptoms, pulmonary function, and markers of inflammation among bar workers before and after a legislative ban on smoking in public places. JAMA 2006;296(14):1742–1748.

Skeer M, Cheng DM, Rigotti NA, Siegel M. Secondhand smoke exposure in the workplace. Am J Prev Med 2005;28(4):331–337.

Trout D, Decker J, Mueller C, Bernert JT, Pirkle J. Exposure of casino employees to environmental tobacco smoke. J Occup Environ Med 1998;40(3):270–276.

Wakefield M, Cameron M, Inglis G, Letcher T, Durkin S. Secondhand smoke exposure and respiratory symptoms among casino, club, and office workers in Victoria, Australia. J Occup Environ Med 2005;47(7):698–703.

Economic Impact

Centers for Disease Control and Prevention. Impact of a smoking ban on restaurant and bar revenues—El Paso, Texas, 2002. MMWR 2004;53(7):150–152. A

Glantz SA. Effect of smokefree bar law on bar revenues in California. Tob Control 2000;9(1):111–112.

Glantz SA, Charlesworth A. Tourism and hotel revenues before and after passage of smoke-free restaurant ordinances. JAMA 1999;281(20):1911–1918.

Glantz SA, Smith LRA. The effect of ordinances requiring smoke-free restaurants and bars on revenues: a follow-up. Am J Public Health 1997;87(10):1687–1693.

Glantz SA, Smith LRA. The effect of ordinances requiring smoke-free restaurants on restaurant sales. Am J Public Health 1994;84(7):1081–1085.

Hyland A, Cummings KM. Restaurant employment before and after the New York City Smoke-Free Air Act. J Public Health Manag Pract 1999;5(1):22–27.

Hyland A, Cummings KM, Nauenberg E. Analysis of taxable sales receipts: was New York City's Smoke-Free Air Act bad for restaurant business? J Public Health Manag Pract 1999;5(1):14–21.

Mandel LL, Alamar BC, Glantz SA. Smoke-free law did not affect revenue from gaming in Delaware. Tob Control 2005;14(1):10–12. A

Pyles MK, Mullineaux DJ, Okoli CTC, Hahn EJ. Economic effect of a smoke-free law in a tobacco-growing community. Tob Control 2007;16(1):66–68. A

Scollo M, Lal A, Hyland A, Glantz S. Review of the quality of studies on the economic effects of smoke-free policies on the hospitality industry. Tob Control 2003;12(1):13–20. A

In addition, the following publications contain examples of all five types of evaluation studies.

ClearWay Minnesota. A toolkit for implementing and defending smoke-free ordinances. Minneapolis, MN: Minnesota Institute of Public Health; 2006. A

New York State Department of Health. The health and economic impact of New York's Clean Indoor Air Act. Albany, NY: New York State Department of Health; 2006.

Notes

Notes

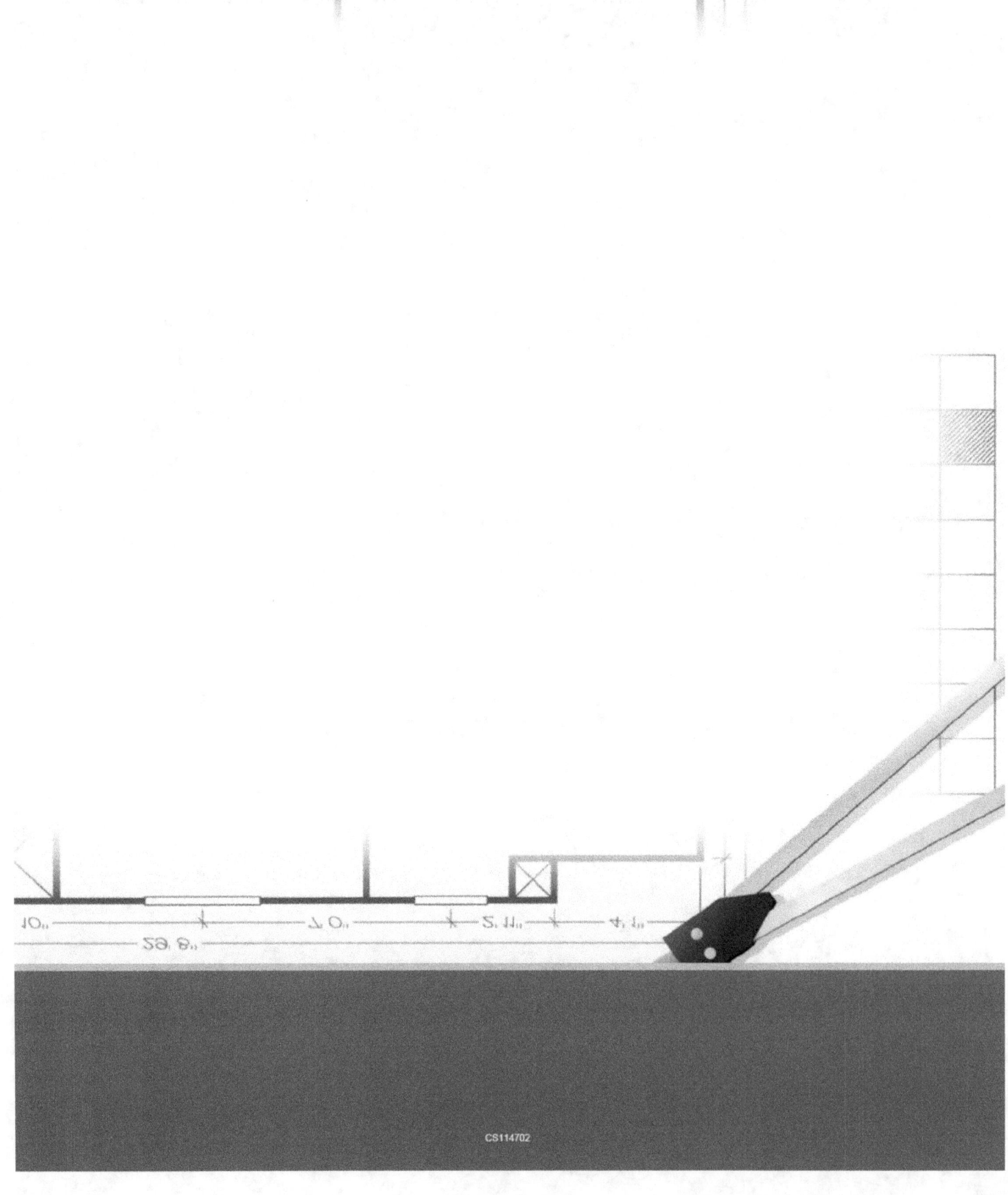